Mathias Roth, Per Henrik Ling

Gymnastic exercises, without apparatus, according to Ling's system

For the due development and strengthening of the human body

Mathias Roth, Per Henrik Ling

Gymnastic exercises, without apparatus, according to Ling's system
For the due development and strengthening of the human body

ISBN/EAN: 9783744736367

Printed in Europe, USA, Canada, Australia, Japan

Cover: Foto ©Lupo / pixelio.de

More available books at **www.hansebooks.com**

GYMNASTIC EXERCISES

WITHOUT APPARATUS,

ACCORDING TO

LING'S SYSTEM,

FOR THE

DUE DEVELOPMENT AND STRENGTHENING OF THE HUMAN BODY.

BY

DR. MATHIAS ROTH,

PHYSICIAN TO PRIVATE MEDICO-GYMNASTIC INSTITUTIONS FOR THE TREATMENT OF
DEFORMITIES AND CHRONIC DISEASES, AT LONDON AND BRIGHTON;
AUTHOR OF SEVERAL WORKS ON EDUCATIONAL AND
MEDICAL GYMNASTICS; ETC.

FIFTH ENLARGED EDITION,

EXTRACTED FROM DR. ROTH'S WORK:

"THE PREVENTION AND CURE OF CHRONIC DISEASES BY MOVEMENTS."

London:

A. N. MYERS & CO.,

15, BERNERS STREET; OXFORD STREET, W.

1876.

TABLE OF CONTENTS.

B 2

APPENDIX.

INTRODUCTION TO THE FIFTH EDITION.

DURING the last twenty-five years, I have tried to introduce the elements of physical education into all elementary, secondary and higher schools. The science of physical education includes the knowledge of the structure and functions of the human body; the knowledge of preserving our health, usually called hygiene; further, the theory and practice of those elementary exercises, which without the use of any external apparatus, are sufficient for the harmonious development of all parts of the human body. Good books on the structure and functions of the human body have been published in sufficient number. Popular books on hygiene are less numerous, and on school hygiene still more scarce.

I therefore tried, about twenty years ago, through the establishment of the Ladies' Sanitary Association, which has hitherto published and distributed more than a million of sanitary tracts, to diminish the prevalent ignorance regarding the preservation of health. The National Health Association lately established on the model of the Ladies' Sanitary Association is also trying to act in the same direction.

As I have seen and am still seeing professionally many deformities and complaints which are mostly caused by ignorance, indifference, and negligence, I felt it my duty as far as it was in the power of a single individual to contribute to the diminution of the complaints I have named, partly by gratuitous courses of instruction to Schoolmistresses who have been theoretically and practically trained in the elements of physical education; and partly by endeavouring, hitherto in vain, to induce the Committee of Council on Education to make elementary physical education an obligatory branch of education in every school, just as reading, writing, and elements of arithmetic.

If the Teachers are paid only for the so-called *three R's*, we cannot expect them to devote their time to physical education, and to give object-lessons on health, on the various parts of the body, and on their use, and to teach how to develop the bodily faculties.

The following Exercises are only an instalment of a single branch of physical education.

No one who has paid any attention to the subject, can doubt that the right use of properly regulated exercises, must have a most beneficial influence on the due development of the human body.

Ling's exercises may be introduced with the greatest advantage into every school and seminary; in fact, they should constitute a part of sound and good education. A healthy body is the best condition for the development of a healthy mind. It is hoped that parents, and all those who are engaged in the noble profession of tuition, will give their earnest attention and their practical support to the enlightened system of Ling.

It need not be said that these exercises are also very useful for preparing the recruit or volunteer for his military training.

Gymnastic games, based on the few exercises described in this pamphlet, are a source of amusement for young and old, in public and private schools, in barracks, in working men's clubs, &c. Persons engaged in sedentary occupations for many hours daily, as clerks, needlewomen, and others, whose stooping position contributes to injure the natural development of the respiratory and abdominal organs, will soon counteract these bad effects, by a daily practice of exercises which call into play all the muscles of the body, without incurring the expenses of gymnastic apparatus.

To enable the blind, the deaf and dumb, and even persons affected mentally, to share in the beneficial effects of rational daily exercise, without exposing them to the danger of being injured, as often happens in exercises with gymnastic apparatus, a series of elementary exercises have been modelled under my superintendence by a first-rate artist; these models have been reproduced in papier-maché, and are sold by the publishers of this pamphlet.

For further information on Scientific, Educational and Medical Gymnastics, I must refer to the works on these subjects, a list of which is given at the end of this pamphlet. Those interested in the practical application of movements for curative and educational purposes, can apply at my Institutions, either here or in Brighton.

In order to make easier the teaching in class of the following exercises, I have added an appendix with 24 figures, which will enable the teacher to attend to a larger number of pupils with more precision and exactitude. A Table of Contents has also been added.

M. ROTH.

48, WIMPOLE STREET, LONDON, W.
28th May, 1876.

GYMNASTIC EXERCISES.

LING'S IDEAS ON THE AIM OF RATIONAL
GYMNASTICS,

AND ON THE INFLUENCE OF MOVEMENTS ON THE DEVELOPMENT AND
STRENGTH OF THE HUMAN BODY.

1. The object to be obtained by Gymnastics, is the harmonious development of the human body by well-defined movements.

2. The body is harmoniously developed when all parts of the body are in the most perfect harmony with each other, and when they are developed as much as the faculties peculiar to the individual admit.

3. Well-defined movements are those which are carefully selected, with regard to the individual to be developed by them.

4. The human body cannot be developed beyond the limits determined by its faculties.

5. Want of exercise may arrest the development, but not destroy the natural faculties.

6. Injurious exercise may prevent the development of our faculties, and thus be injurious to the harmony of the bodily development.

7. Stiffness or immobility of some parts of the body, in young persons, is usually caused by too much strength of those parts, and is compensated by weakness of other parts.

8. Too much strength of one part will be lessened, and insufficient strength of another will be increased, by exercise equally distributed all over the body.

9. The strength or weakness of a single individual does not depend upon the large or small volume, but upon the relative proportions of the various parts of his body.

10. Health and the maximum of strength, depend upon the harmonious development of all parts of the body.

11. The faculty of moving the body with precision, energy, and during a definite period of time, is of the greatest importance for everybody, but especially for those whose duty it is to defend the country, as they are obliged to move, and to overcome many impediments, while burdened with weapons, accoutrements, and baggage.

12. To be able to obtain and preserve the maximum of strength, we must accustom ourselves to positions in which the powers of breathing and moving are least interfered with ; because the power of moving depends, to a great extent, upon the power of breathing.

13. The present practice of exercising the limbs only, is not sufficient for obtaining the final results of rational Gymnastics; and the power of using well the arms and legs depends, not only upon the strength of those limbs, but also upon that of all other parts of the body.

14. Persons who are well trained in Gymnastic Exercises, bear with more ease all kinds of bodily fatigue, and the changes of temperature and climate; they are generally in good spirits, and perform all their movements with a sensation of ease.

15. The movements selected at the commencement for physical training are very simple, and their execution is easy ; by degrees, and without the least danger of any injurious effect, the most difficult movements are made use of; the persons who are trained are aware of the increase of their strength, and become conscious of the amount of work and exercise they might be able to go through.

A FEW RULES FOR THE PRACTICE OF THE ELEMENTARY EXERCISES.

1. The exercises are divided according to the principal parts of the body, viz., into those of the arms, legs, head, and trunk ; but as all these parts must be in perfect harmony, it is *not* indifferent whether we practise only certain movements.

2. In the beginning, the positions are to be practised.

3. No movement is to be done with any strain.

4. The action of breathing must not be stopped during the exercises.

5. The best dress is a loose one, and for ladies a blouse (*vide* figure), without stays or bustles, which are soon superfluous, if the following exercises are well and moderately practised.

6. The movements of the head and trunk are to be done slowly ; also those of the legs, by which the body is raised or lowered ; if the strength and flexibility increase, these movements must be executed *very slowly.*

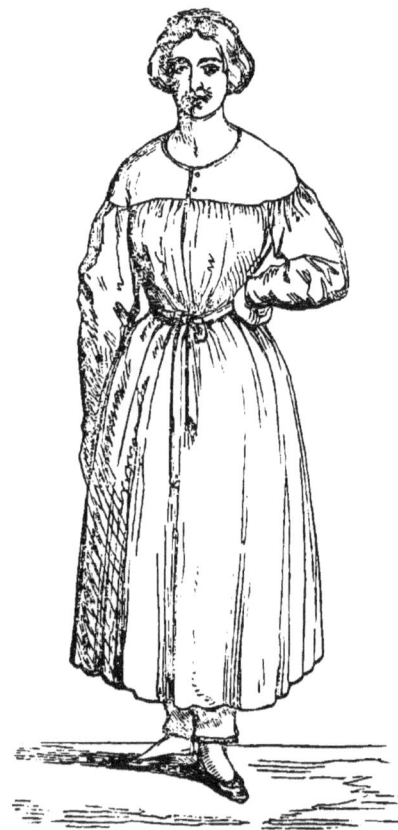

7. The movements of the arms are to be done quickly, and the more quickly they are performed, the more strength is developed.

8. The movements vary, and one and the same movement is not to be repeated more than two or three times in succession.

9. The movements, although they are changed, must not be executed only and principally with one part, which would then become stronger than all the others, and thus interfere with the harmony of the body.

10. The exercises are performed by healthy persons according to the numeric order of the tables of exercises. We should not proceed to any following table, before we have well practised the exercises of the preceding one.

11. Between the single exercises, an interval of half a minute to two minutes is desirable.

12. Not more than ten to twelve exercises should be practised at the same time each day.

13. Persons who are indisposed, or who complain of one part being weaker than another, should consult a medical man acquainted with the effects of movements, as to which if any, should be used, exercises being sometimes injurious.

14. The following exercises are called FREE Exercises, because they are executed without the help of any gymnastic apparatus.

ADVANTAGES OF FREE EXERCISES.

Their great advantage consists in this:—

1. That the movements being very simple, are easily understood and easily executed.

2. Much time is saved, because they can be executed simultaneously by many persons.

3. The expense of apparatus and machines is saved, and the dress is less spoiled.

4. The free exercises can be executed in any place; in the open air as well as in-doors, in schools, barracks, in the open field, in the camp, and in the bivouac.

5. As every motion of a free exercise is to be executed exactly, and, if there are many persons going through the exercises, they act simultaneously, all must accustom themselves to a certain amount of attention and precision, by which means the sense of order is developed, and the attention sharpened.

6. The free exercises produce an agreeable sensation during all the movements, and develop, better than the exercises on gymnastic apparatus, a good posture of the body, and an appropriate appearance and deportment in ordinary life.

COMMENCING, IMMEDIATE, AND FINAL POSITIONS.

Every gymnastic movement used for the harmonious development of the body, being a definite movement, has a *definite form*.

Every definite form has a definite point in which it begins, and this is called the *Commencing Position*.

All the positions in which the body, or a part of it, is placed between the commencing and final position, are called *Intermediate Positions*.

The position in which the moved body, or part of the body, returns to the state of rest, is the *Final Position*.

TIME, AND WORD OF COMMAND.

All the exercises composed of different movements, are divided into different spaces of time, during which a certain movement is executed; these divisions of time are called *Motions*, and are indicated by " one, two," &c.

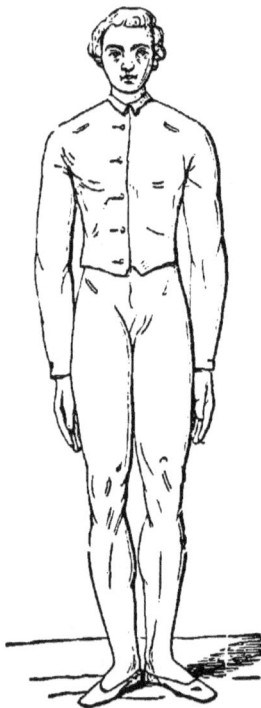

The exercises are executed at word of command. The command consists of two parts : the first is called *Attention*, and the second *Execution*. For instance, in " RIGHT FOOT FORWARDS: PLACE!" the three first words form the first part and stand before the colon (:); they call the attention to an action for which the right foot is to be prepared; but, only when the word of *Execution*, " PLACE!" is given, the movement of placing the right foot forwards is executed.

FIRST POSITION. (FIG. II.)

This is also called the *Fundamenta Position*. The word of command is Position! or RECTANGULAR POSITION.

Fig. II.

FEET : OPEN !

The heels are in a line, and closed; the knees straight, well stretched, and so turned outwards, that the feet may form a right angle between the heels; the arms are well stretched, and close to the sides of the erect body ; the elbows directed backwards; the wrists touch the outer sides of the thighs; the fingers, close to each other, with the thumb in front, are stretched in a straight line ; the head straight—the eyes directed forwards; the chest projects, while the hips are kept slightly backwards, and almost in a line with the ankle-joints.

SECOND POSITION. (FIG. III.)

FEET : CLOSE !

The feet being in the first position; at ONE ! the toes are slightly raised; at TWO ! the legs and feet are turned towards each other; at THREE! the toes are placed down. These three motions are executed very quickly, and thus they form apparently only one motion.

FEET : OPEN !

At ONE! the toes are raised ; at TWO ! the legs and feet are turned outwards; at THREE ! the feet being in a right angle, the toes are placed down. These three motions, being quickly executed, form apparently only one motion.

FEET ALTERNATELY OPEN AND CLOSE !

Is an exercise based on the two preceding positions, in which the feet are alternately opened and closed, at ONE! TWO! ONE! TWO! till HALT is ordered, when the first position is resumed.

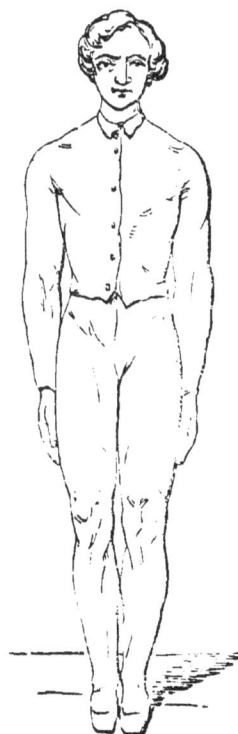

Fig. III.

POSITIONS WITH DISTANCE.

The length of the pupil's foot is the measure, called *One Distance;* two distances between the heels, in a lateral, or in a front or rear direction, are sufficient for girls and women; for boys and men, three, and sometimes even four distances are chosen.

WALK POSITIONS

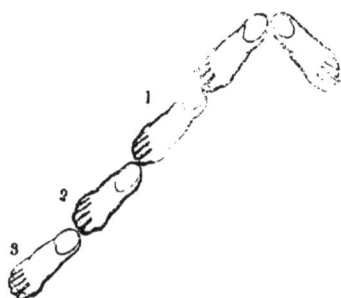

Fig. IV.

Are those in which one foot is placed either forwards or backwards, at *one* distance from the heel of the other foot, the commencing positions being Feet Open! the word of command RIGHT (or left) FOOT FORWARDS (or backwards): PLACE!—At PLACE! the right foot is placed forwards, and retains the rectangular direction of the commencing position. (*See* Fig. IV., 1.)

STRAIGHT WALK POSITIONS.

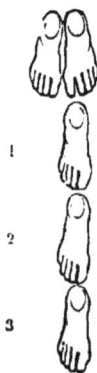

Fig. V.

These are, with regard to the distance, similar to the previous; but differ, *First,* in the commencing position being FEET: CLOSE! and *Secondly,* the foot to be moved being placed in the *same* line with the other. (*See* Fig. V., 1.) The command is, RIGHT (left) FOOT STRAIGHT FORWARDS (or backwards): PLACE!—At POSITION! the foot which was placed either forwards or backwards is replaced into the commencing position; at FEET: CHANGE! the other foot is placed into *straight walk position,* either forwards or backwards, according to the word of command.

FEET ALTERNATELY FORWARDS (or backwards): PLACE !

Is an exercise based on *walk position.* At ONE ! the foot is replaced into the commencing positions ; at Two ! the other foot is placed into the position commanded.

The alternate positions are continued till HALT is given, when the commencing position is taken up.

FEET ALTERNATELY STRAIGHT FORWARDS (or backwards): PLACE !

Is an exercise similar to the preceding, but FEET: CLOSE ! is the *commencing* position.

PASS POSITIONS. (FIG. VI.)

Are those in which one foot is placed either forwards or backwards, at *two* (three or more) distances from the heel of the other foot; the commencing positions are either FEET: OPEN ! or FEET: CLOSE !

Fig. V. A.

The words of command are, RIGHT, (or left) FOOT TWO (three) DISTANCES FORWARDS (or backwards): PLACE !

At PLACE ! the right foot is placed forwards, and retains the direction of the commencing position. (*See* Figs. IV. and V., 2 or 3 ; also the position of the feet in Fig. V. A.)

The upper part of the body is in a line with the left (right) leg, which is well stretched, while the left foot remains firmly on the floor; the right (left) knee is bent, and almost perpendicular over the right (left) toes; the body and left leg are inclined, and form an angle of about forty-five degrees, with

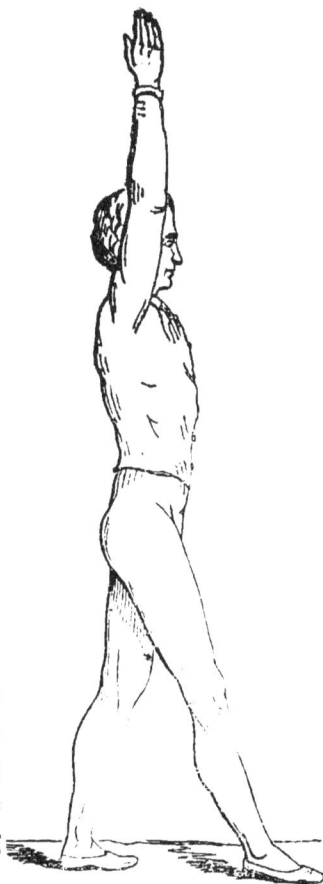

the horizontal floor; the head is in a line with the right (left)
knees and toes. (Fig. VI. represents the left *pass position*
with *heels raised.*)

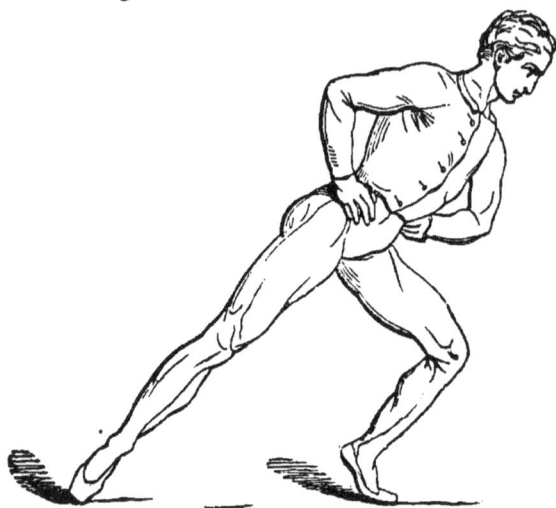

Fig. VI.

STRAIGHT PASS POSITION.

Is similar to the preceding, but the commencing position is
FEET: CLOSE!

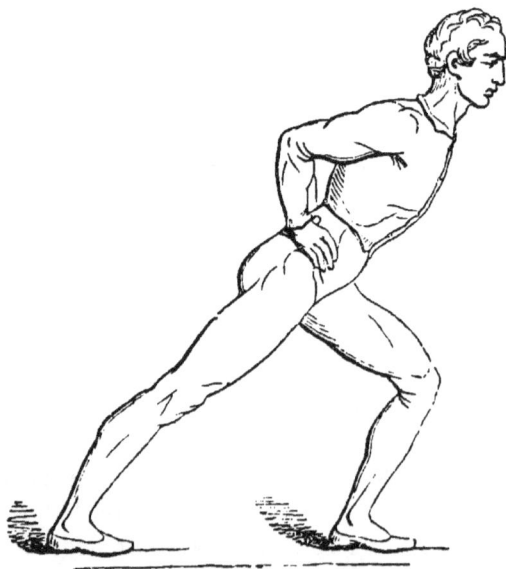

RIGHT (or left) FOOT TWO (or three) DISTANCES STRAIGHT FORWARDS :
PLACE !

See Fig. V., 2 (or 3), and Fig. VII., which shows the position of the body and head.

FEET ALTERNATELY TWO (or three) DISTANCES FORWARDS : PLACE !

The preceding position is executed at FEET: CHANGE ! in two motions. At ONE ! the front foot is replaced into the commencing position : at TWO ! the other foot is placed forwards.

STRIDE POSITIONS.

FEET SIDEWAYS ONE (two, three) DISTANCES : PLACE !

Commencing positions are FEET: OPEN ! or FEET : CLOSE ! (Fig. VIII., and Fig. IX.) In two motions.

At ONE ! the left foot is placed to the left, *half* a distance from, and in a straight line with the right foot, which, at TWO ! is placed to the right another half a distance. The space between the heels is equal to the length of the pupil's foot; the knee is stretched, and the body erect, while the feet are placed sideways, and retain the direction of the commencing position (Fig. X.)

The commencing position is resumed at POSITION !—and at ONE ! the left foot is

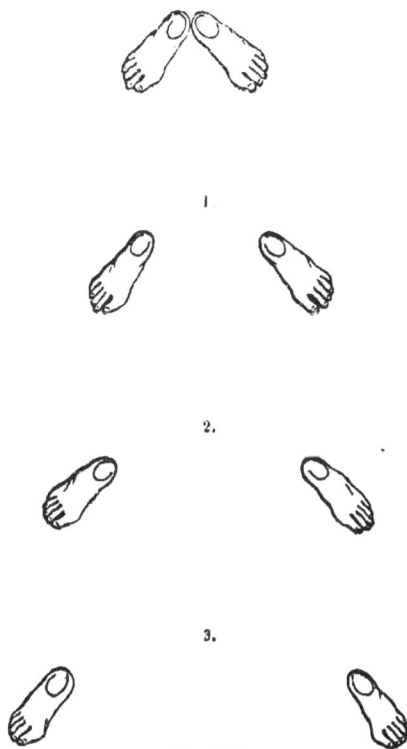

Fig. VIII.

C

placed at half a distance towards the right foot, which, at Two!
is placed near the left; if the feet are to be placed apart at
two or three distances, each foot is placed sideways at one
half of the distance which is ordered; for girls, two distances
only are commanded.   Figs. VIII. and IX., illustrate the
position of the feet when placed apart, either in the position
FEET: CLOSE! (Fig. IX.) or FEET: OPEN! (Fig. VIII.)

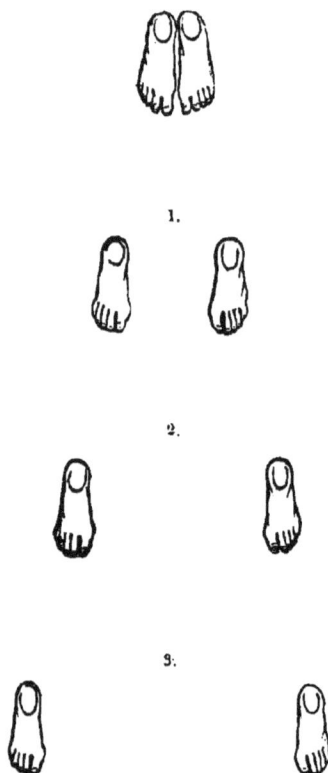

Fig. IX.

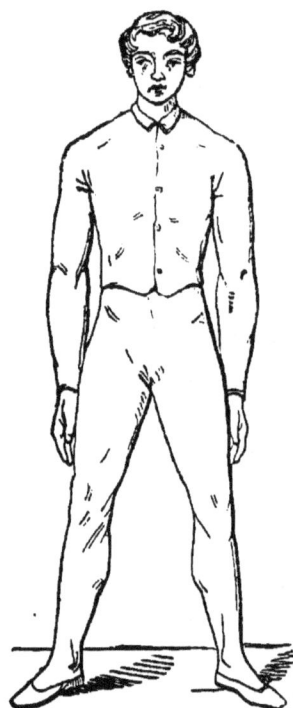

Fig. X.

STRIDE STANDING POSITION.

BALANCING POSITIONS (Fig. XI.)

Are those in which the body rests on one foot only, or only on
a part of the foot, viz., on the front part of the foot, on the
toes, or on the heels.   Only advanced pupils make use of these
positions.   Fig. XI. shows also stretch position of the arms.

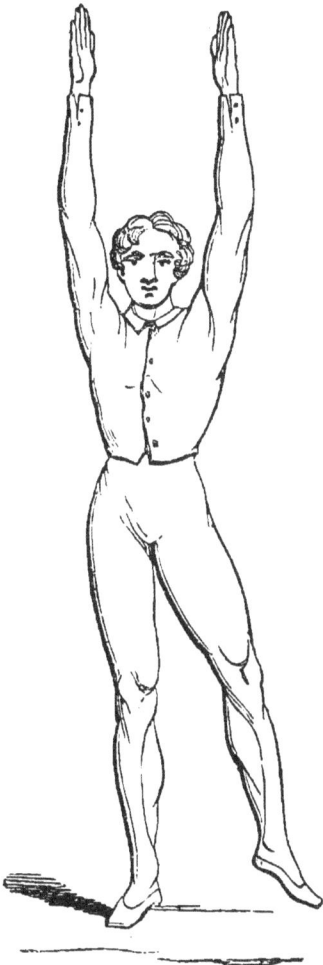

Fig. XII.

Fig. XI.

STRETCH RIGHT BALANCING POSITION.

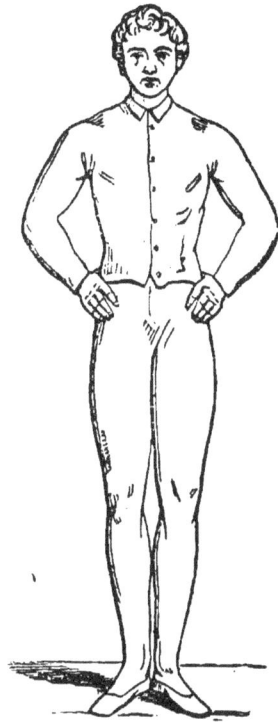

HIPS : FIRM ! (FIG. XII.)

The forearms are smartly raised, and the palms of the hands placed firmly on the hips, with the thumbs backwards; the forefinger on the edge of the hip-bone, the elbows in a line with the body, and the shoulders are kept down and backwards. This *position* serves as a *support* to the body, and enables us to retain with more ease the upright position, while various exercises of the legs and of the trunk are executed, or when balancing and other difficult positions are chosen.

c 2

MOVEMENTS OF THE HEAD.

All movements of the head are executed in *slow* time ; th
elementary movements are *Turning* and *Bending* of the heac.
Walk or stride positions, with the hips firm, are suitable
commencing positions for beginners; the pass and balancing
positions can be used by those who are more advanced.
Attention must be paid that—

1. The body should remain in the vertical position.

2. The shoulders and hips should not be turned, but
remain square.

3. That neither of the shoulders should be raised or
lowered, during the bending of the head to the side.

4. That the feet should remain in the commencing position.

5. That the body should rest equally on both legs, which
should be well stretched, in stride or in walk position.

1. TURNING OF THE HEAD.

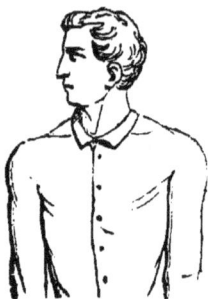

Fig. XIII.

(*a*) Head right: Turn! Forwards:
Turn !

(*b*) Head left: Turn! Forwards :
Turn ! Position!

The head, without being *bent* to
any side, is slowly and horizontally
turned to the right (or left), till the
chin is over the shoulder.

At FORWARDS: TURN! the head
is turned forwards, as in the fundamental position.

2. BENDING OF THE HEAD.

This is also called HEAD FLEXION.

(*a*) Head forwards: Bend ! Stretch !
(*b*) Head backwards : Bend ! Stretch !
(*c*) Head to the right: Bend ! Stretch !
(*d*) Head to the left: Bend ! Stretch !

At the order, HEAD FORWARDS:
BEND! (Fig. XIV.) the head, which
is held straight, without being in
the least turned to one side, is
slowly bent forwards until the chin
slightly touches the chest.   The
upper part of the body, especially
the shoulders, must be held firm.

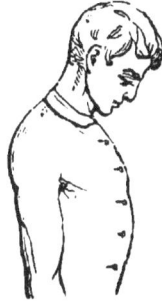

At STRETCH! the head is raised
as in the fundamental position. Both

Fig. XIV.

movements are done steadily, and not by jerks.

At HEAD BACKWARDS: BEND!
(Fig. XV.) the head, without being
turned or bent sideways, is slowly
bent backwards; at STRETCH! it
is raised into the previous position.
The head is neither to be bent too
far backwards, nor to be retained
more than a few seconds in this
position.   ·

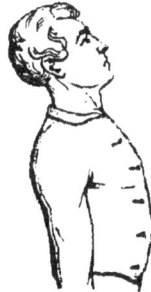

Fig. XV.

At HEAD TO THE RIGHT (or left):
BEND! (Fig. XVI.) the head is slowly
bent to the right (left) side; neither
the face nor the shoulders are to be
turned; the raising of the shoulder
opposite to the side towards which
the head bends, and the lowering
of the shoulder on the side to
which the bending is made, must be
prevented.

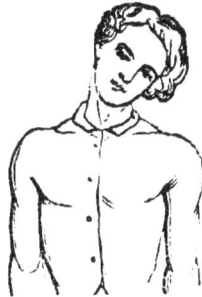

Fig. XVI.

3. TURNING OF THE HEAD ALTERNATELY TO
BOTH SIDES.

HEAD RIGHT AND LEFT: TURN!

4. BENDING OF THE HEAD ALTERNATELY EITHER
   FORWARDS AND BACKWARDS, OR TO THE
   RIGHT AND LEFT.

HEAD FORWARDS AND BACKWARDS : BEND !
HEAD TO THE RIGHT AND LEFT : BEND !

These movements of the head are done first towards one,
and then, without the intermediate order of STRETCH, to the
opposite direction.

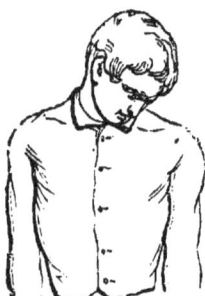

Fig. XVII.

5. BENDING OF THE HEAD
   WHILE IT IS TURNED TO
   ONE SIDE.

   (FIG. XVII.)

   HEAD LEFT (or right) : TURN !
   FORWARDS BEND ! STRETCH !
   BACKWARDS BEND ! STRETCH !

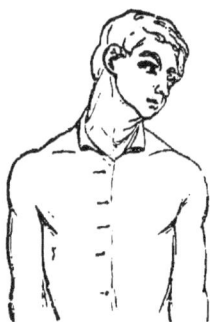

Fig. XVIII.

6. TURNING OF THE HEAD
   WHILE IT IS BENT.

   (FIG. XVIII.)

   Head to the right (or left) : Bend !
   Head to the right : Turn !
   Head to the left : Turn !
   Head backwards : Bend !
   Head to the left (right) : Turn !

MOVEMENTS OF THE EYES.

These movements are done in slow time. All standing
positions are used as commencing positions. The words of
command are :—

1. EYES : to the right. 2. To the left. 3. To the right,
and up. 4. To the left, and down. 5. T

the left, and up. 7. To the right, and down. 8. From the right to the left, and *vice versâ*, in a horizontal line. 9. From the left to the right, in half a circle.

The usual faults are—

1. The head is turned, bent, or raised, to the side to which the eyes are moved.

2. The forehead is frowning when the eyes are directed upwards.

3. When the eyes are moved from one side to the other, they move in a circular instead of a straight line.

MOVEMENTS OF THE ARMS

Are executed quickly, and each movement repeated three or four times. The commencing positions are all *walk, stride, pass,* and *balancing* positions.

STRETCHING OF THE ARMS IN THE FIVE PRINCIPAL DIRECTIONS.

The stretching of the arms refers especially to the elbow-joint, which must be bent before it is stretched. The words of command for this preparatory exercise are,

I. ARMS UPWARDS: BEND!
(Fig. XIX. *a*.)

The upper arm is immoveable, and close to the side of the body, while the elbow is bent, and the forearm placed in front of the upper arm; the shoulders and elbows are well drawn down; the hands are bent at the wrists, without being stiff; while the tips of the fingers, which are bent and close to each other, touch the armpits.

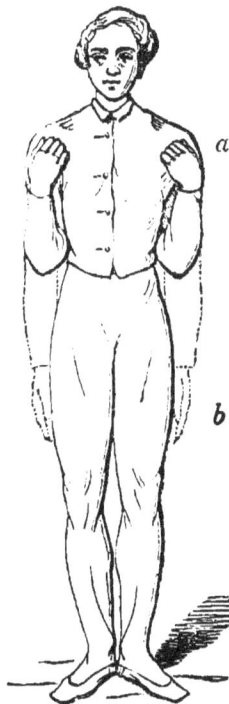

Fig. XIX.

The usual faults, which must be avoided, during this exercise are—

1. The elbows are not placed as low as required.

2. The upper arms are not placed firmly, and sufficiently near to the side of the body.

3. The wrist and fingers are kept stiff, and do not touch the armpits.

II. ARMS DOWNWARDS : STRETCH !

(Fig. XIX. *b*.)

The fingers and forearms are stretched, and brought down into the fundamental position, with the thumb in front.

The words of command for the movements of the arms are—

Arms upwards : Stretch ! ⎫
Arms sideways : Stretch ! ⎬ One !
Arms forwards : Stretch ! ⎬ Two !
Arms backwards ! Stretch ! ⎭
Arms downwards : Stretch !

All these movements are executed in two motions.

At ONE ! the arms are bent upwards.

At TWO ! the arms are stretched, and the hands and fingers placed in a straight line with the arms.

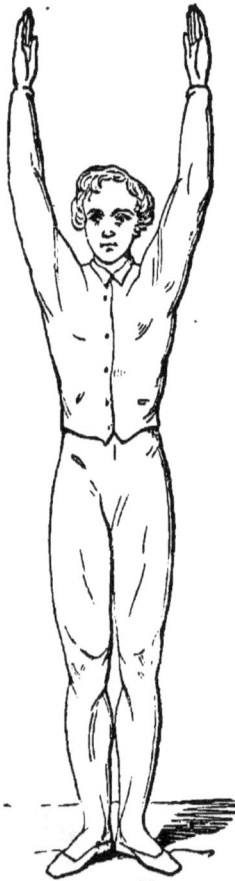

ARMS UPWARDS : STRETCH !

(Fig. XX.)

At ONE ! ARMS UPWARDS : BEND !

At TWO ! the arms, hands, and fingers are well stretched upwards and parallel to each other, and are placed vertically, as near as possible to the head, which remains immoveable : the hands are facing each other during the movement, the fingers close to each other, and the little finger in front.

Fig. XX.

ARMS SIDEWAYS STRETCH.　(Fig. XXI.)

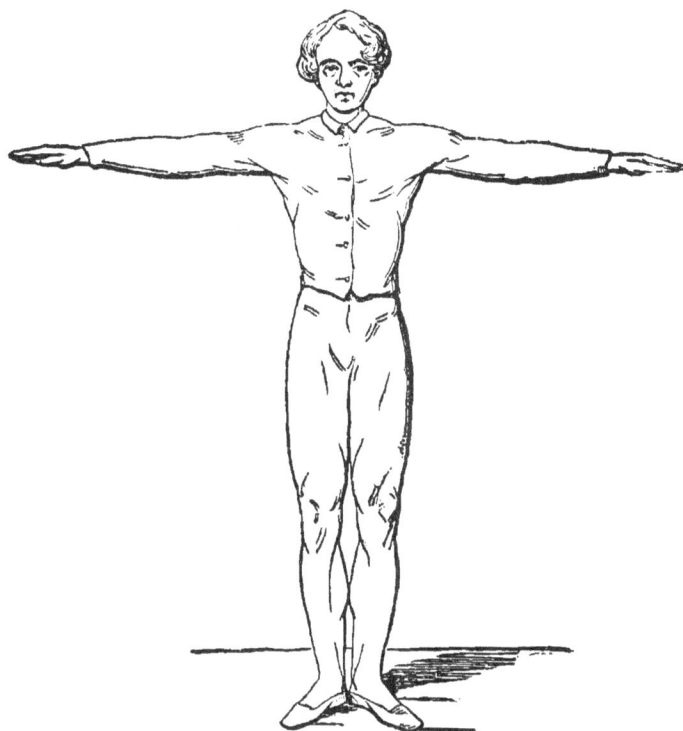

Fig. XXI.

At One! Arms upwards: Bend!

At Two! the arms, hands, and fingers are quickly stretched sideways, at the height of, and in a line with the shoulders, which are well drawn downwards and backwards; the shoulder-blades are placed as near to each other as is practicable without producing pain; the middle finger should be in a straight line with the middle of the highest point of the shoulder; the thumb in front, and the knuckles inclined upwards.

ARMS FORWARDS: STRETCH!　(Fig. XXII.)

At One! Arms upwards: Bend!

At Two! the arms, hands, and fingers are stretched

horizontally forwards; the arms are parallel to each other, and in a line with the shoulders, which are well drawn downwards and backwards; the palms face each other, the thumbs are upwards, and the fingers close to each other.

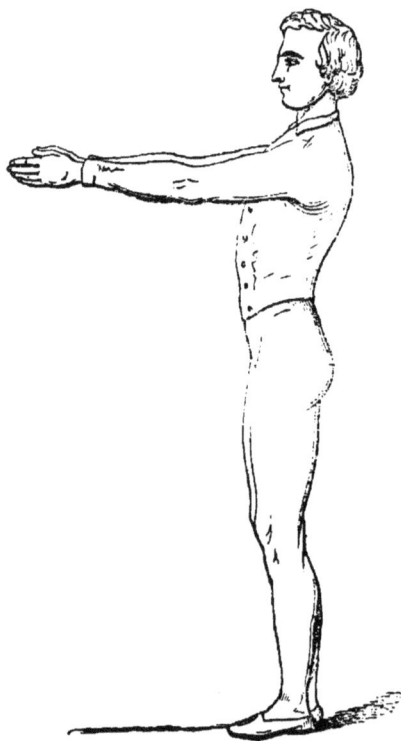 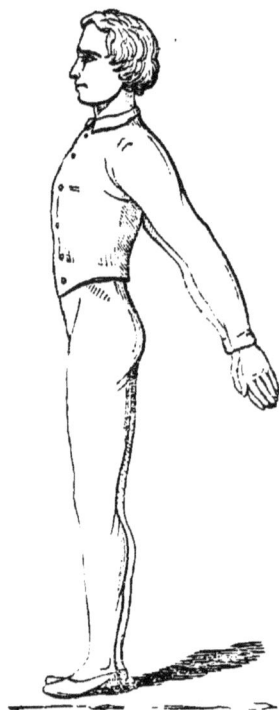

Fig. XXII.   Fig. XXIII.

ARMS BACKWARDS: STRETCH! (Fig. XXIII.)

At One! Arms upwards: Bend!

At Two! the arms, hands, and fingers, are well and quickly stretched backwards; the body is immoveable, the shoulders down and back; the palms face each other, the fingers are close to each other, the little finger is upwards.

ARMS DOWNWARDS : STRETCH !

At One! Arms upwards: Bend!

At Two! the forearms, hands, and fingers, are stretched downwards near the body, while the upper arms remain immoveable.

The most frequent *faults* during the movements of the arms are—

1. That the body is not steady and firm, but moves in the direction towards which the exercise is to be done.

2. The shoulders are not kept sufficiently firmly backwards and downwards.

3. The arms are not parallel to each other while stretched forwards or upwards, and while stretching upwards they are not vertical, and not sufficiently near to the side of the head.

STRETCHING OF THE ARMS HORIZONTALLY IN
DIFFERENT DIRECTIONS.

One ! Arms upwards : Bend !
Two ! Right (left) arm forwards, and
       Left (right) arm sideways : Stretch !
Arms : Change !
One ! Arms upwards : Bend !
Two ! Left (right) arm forwards, and
       Right (left) arms sideways : Stretch !
At Position ! and
One ! Arms upwards : Bend !
Two ! Arms downwards : Stretch !

STRETCHING OF THE ARMS VERTICALLY IN
DIFFERENT DIRECTIONS.

One ! Arms upwards : Bend !
Two ! Right (left) arm upwards, and
       Left (right) arm downwards (or backwards): Stretch !

Arms : Change ! One ! Two ! } Are executed in a way similar to the preced-
Position ! One ! Two ! } ing, only the direction of the arms is different.

STRETCHING OF THE ARMS ALTERNATELY IN DIFFERENT DIRECTIONS.

The words of command are —

1. Right (left) arm upwards, and
   Left (right) arm sideways :
2. Right (left) arm upwards, and
   Left (right) arm forwards :
3. Right (left) arm upwards, and
   Left (right) arm backwards :

Stretch !
One !
Two !

Arms :
Change !
One ! Two !
Position !
One ! Two !

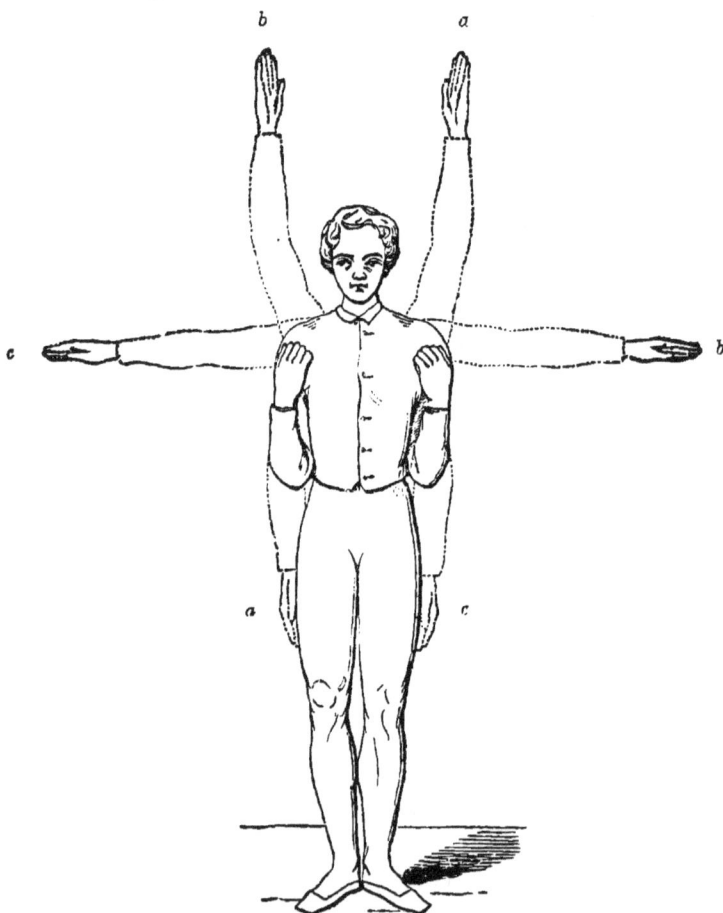

Fig. XXIV.

Fig. XXIV., *aa, bb, cc,,* illustrates three different positions, with the arms in different directions.

At STRETCH! and ONE! the arms are bent upwards. At TWO! the arms are stretched as ordered.

At ARMS: CHANGE! and ONE! the arms are bent upwards. At TWO! each arm is placed in the position the other was in before.

At POSITION! and ONE! the arms are bent upwards. At TWO! they are stretched down.

BENDING AND STRETCHING OF THE FOREARMS,

ARMS HALF FORWARDS : BEND! SIDEWAYS : STRETCH !

At BEND! the upper arms are quickly raised sideways, to a level with the shoulders, and simultaneously the forearms bent in a forward direction at RIGHT angles with the upper arms ; hand and fingers well stretched, the palms facing each other.

At BACKWARDS: STRETCH! the forearms are thrown back into a STRAIGHT line with the upper arms, which are kept immoveable in their position sideways, so that both arms are in a line with the body.

ARMS FORWARDS : BEND !
SIDEWAYS : STRETCH !

This exercise is similar to the preceding.

At BEND! the forearm is, however, laid along the upper arm, till the thumb touches the outer and upper part of the chest, while

At STRETCH! the forearms are thrown out till in a line with the upper arm, which remains immoveable.

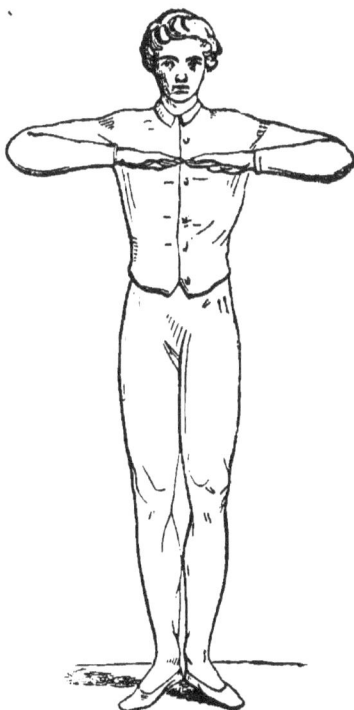

Fig. XXV.

ARMS FULLY FORWARDS : BEND ! BACKWARDS : STRETCH !
(FIG. XXV.)

At BEND ! the arms are bent at the elbows as in the preceding exercise; the forearms are brought forwards till the tips of the fingers meet, in front of and near the upper part of the chest.

AT STRETCH ! the arms are stretched briskly as FAR BACK as the shoulder-joints permit; the horizontal position of the arms is retained.

The forearm movements can also be executed, while the commencing position is different for each arm ; for instance—

Right arm half forwards : }
Left arm forwards :   } Bend ! Sideways : Stretch ! or,

Left arms half forwards : } Bend! Left sideways: Stretch !
Right arm fully forwards: } and Right backwards: Stretch !

TURNING OF THE HANDS.

Fig. XXVI.
One.

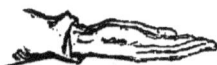

XXVII.
Two.

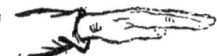

XXVIII.
Three.

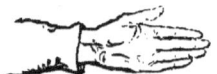

XXIX.
Four.

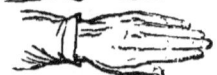

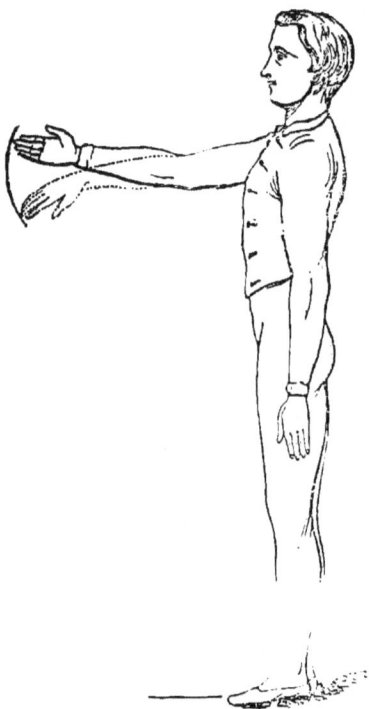

Fig. XXX.

The commencing positions are ARMS FORWARDS (or sideways) : STRETCH ! HANDS ! TURN !

At ONE ! the hands are turned outwards, with the back of the hand down.

At TWO ! the hands are turned inwards, with the back of the hand up.

At THREE ! the hands are turned partly outwards, with

the back of the hand outwards, the thumb up, and the little finger down.

At FOUR! the hands are turned with the palm of the hand outwards, the thumb down, the little finger up.

Fig. XXX. shows the way the forearm is moved, while the upper arm is steady.

MOVEMENTS OF THE TRUNK

Are done in slow time. For beginners, the walk or stride positions are suitable commencing positions. Those who are more advanced can choose pass, straight pass, and balancing positions, combined with different positions of the arms.

BENDING OF THE TRUNK FORWARDS AND

BACKWARDS.

HIPS: FIRM! TRUNK FORWARDS:

BEND! STRETCH!

At BEND! the trunk is gently bent at the lowest part of the spine, without twisting the body or moving the head, which remains in a line with the trunk. The face inclines slightly downwards, the legs and knees are firm.

At STRETCH! the trunk returns to the erect position.

If the trunk is bent forwards while the arms are stretched upwards, the face is opposite the knees, and the hands touch the toes, as seen in Fig. XXXII., *a*. It is essential that the knees should remain stretched.

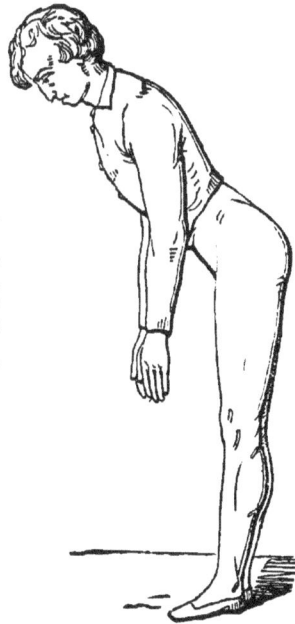

Fig. XXXI.

INCLINATION OF THE TRUNK

Is a movement in the hip-joints, by which the upper part of the body is inclined forwards without bending the spine.

The Figs. XXXI. and XXXII. *b*, represent the inclination, and the dotted lines *aa*, the bending of the trunk.

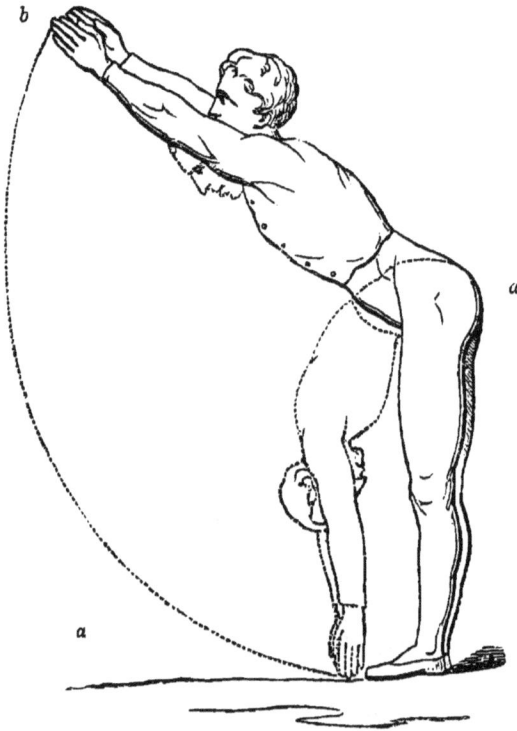

Fig. XXXII.

TRUNK BACKWARDS : BEND ! STRE̅

(Fig. XXXIII.)

The trunk bends gently backwards, the   lirected slightly upwards.

At STRETCH ! the previous position is re̅

In Fig. XXXIII. A, the commencing position is a walking position, with the left arm on the hip, and the right stretched up, the right foot in straight walk position.

Fig. XXXIII. B, is trunk bending backwards, with both arms stretched upwards, and the right foot in walk position.

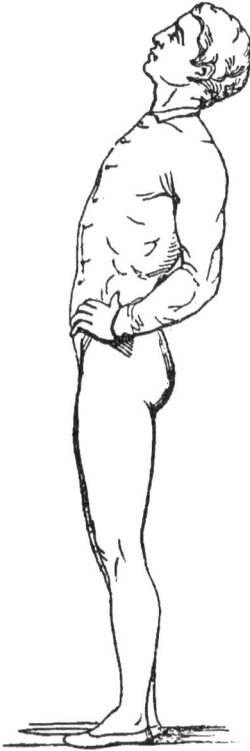 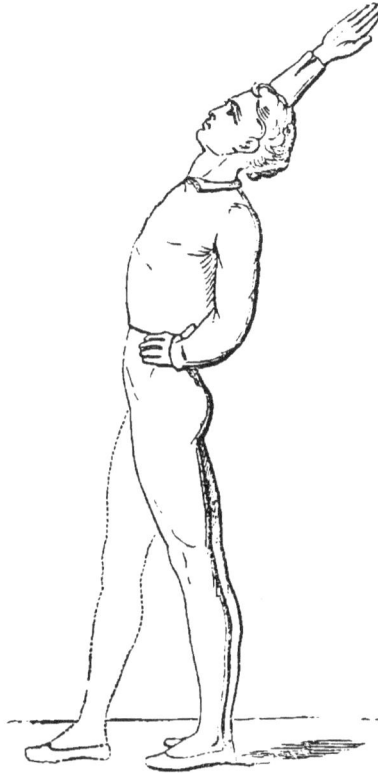

Fig. XXXIII.   Fig. XXXIII. A.

BENDING OF THE TRUNK SIDEWAYS. (*See* FIG. XXXIV.)

TRUNK TO THE RIGHT (left): BEND! STRETCH!

At BEND! the trunk is bent to the right (left), as far as it is possible without raising the left (right) foot from the ground; the head in a line with the trunk, the legs unyielding. The arms hang freely down, and the hands accommodate themselves to the movement, the right (left) by sliding down the right (left) thigh to the knee; the left (right) by sliding up the left (right)

D

thigh to the hip.   The upper part of the body is not to be twisted.

At STRETCH! the body is slowly and steadily raised into the erect position.

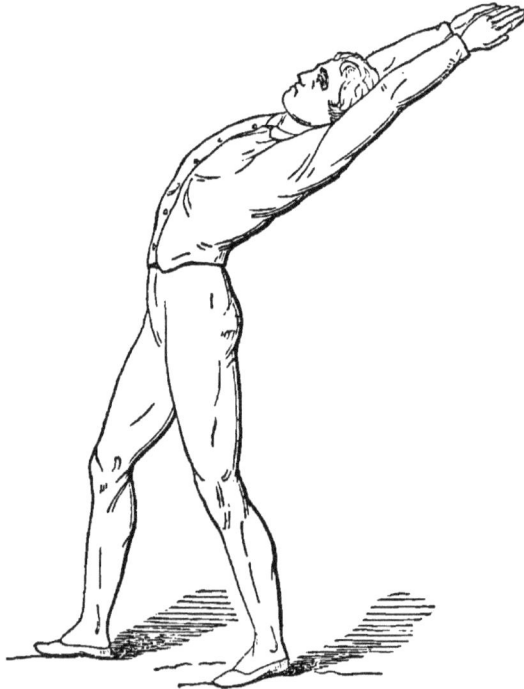

Fig. XXXIII. B.

BENDING OF THE TRUNK TO THE RIGHT AND LEFT ALTERNATELY.
(*See* FIG. XXXIV.)

Trunk to the right: Bend!

Trunk to the left: Bend! Stretch!

The movement from the right to the left and in the opposite direction, is done without stopping.

TURNING OF THE TRUNK.

Consists in twisting the upper part of the body round its longitudinal axis, and above the hips.

TRUNK TO THE RIGHT: TURN!   FORWARDS: TURN.
(FIG. XXXV.)

The body is twisted steadily to the right side, till the shoulders are at a right angle with the front line; thus the fourth part of a circle is described by each shoulder. The head, preserving its original position with regard to the trunk, moves simultaneously with the trunk ; after a short pause, at TRUNK FORWARDS : TURN! the trunk is steadily brought into the previous position.

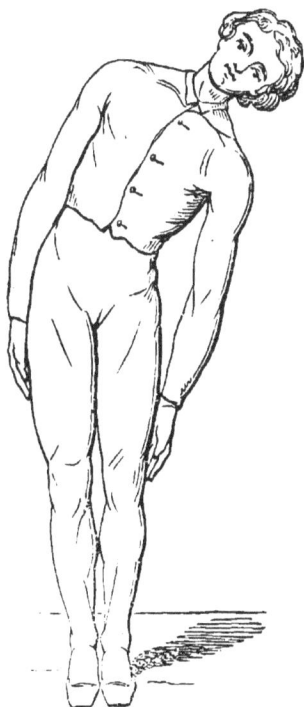

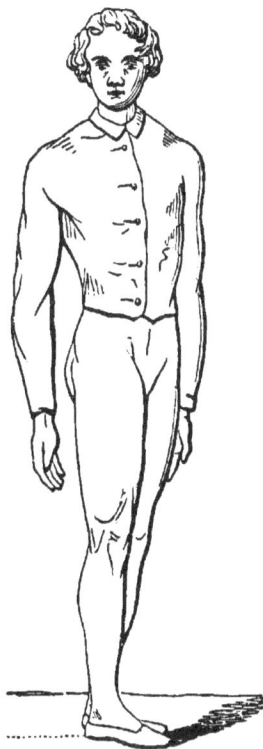

Fig. XXXIV.   Fig. XXXV.

At TRUNK TO THE LEFT: TURN! FORWARDS: TURN! the movement is done first to the left, and, after a short pause, forwards.

TURNING OF THE TRUNK TO THE RIGHT ,AND LEFT ALTERNATELY.

TRUNK TO THE RIGHT AND LEFT : TURN!

The movement from the right to the left, and in the opposite direction, is done without stopping.

2 D

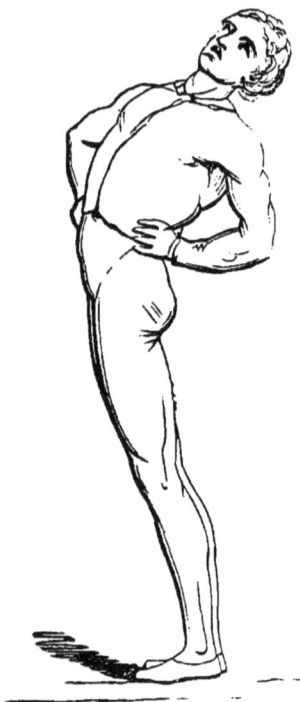

Fig. XXXVI.

BENDING OF THE TRUNK BACK-
WARDS WHILE TURNED TO THE
LEFT (OR RIGHT.)

(FIG. XXXVI.)

Commencing position is—

Hips: Firm!
Trunk to the right (or
left): Turn!
The bending is done at
Backwards: Bend!
At, Stretch! and Trunk
forwards: Turn! the fun-
damental position is re-
sumed.

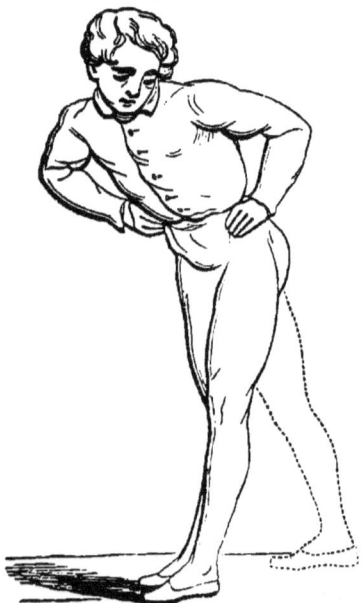

BENDING OF THE TRUNK FOR-
WARDS WHILE IT IS TURNED
TO THE LEFT (OR RIGHT.)

(FIG. XXXVII.)

Commencing position is—

Hips: Firm!
Trunk to the right (or
left): Turn!

Words of command are—

TRUNK FORWARDS: BEND!
STRETCH!
TRUNK FORWARDS: TURN!

LEG AND FOOT MOVEMENTS

Can be done either in slow or quick time. The commencing positions are FEET: OPEN! or FEET: CLOSE! and the various *walk*, *pass*, and *balancing* positions, can also be combined with various positions of the arms and body.

RAISING OF THE BODY ON THE TOES.

(FIG. XXXVIII.)

Heels: Raise! Sink! One! Two! (repeat.)

At RAISE! the heels are slowly raised while the body remains erect, the feet still remaining in the commencing position, with the heels close to each other. The body is, during a few seconds, in the raised position.

At SINK! the heels and body are slowly and gently lowered.

This balancing exercise can be practised in the following commencing positions:—

(*a*) Feet sideways: Place! Heels: Raise! Sink! &c.

(*b*) Right (left) foot forwards: Place! Heels: Raise! Sink!

(*c*) Feet: Close! Heels: Raise! &c.

(*d*) Feet: Close! Right (left) foot forwards: Place! Heels: Raise! &c.

Fig. XXXVIII.

These exercises are also combined with arm movements in such a manner, that the heels are raised, and the arms simultaneously stretched, or the arms are bent while the body sinks on the heels.

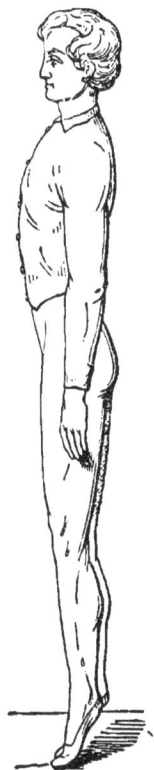

BENDING AND STRETCHING OF THE KNEES.

(FIG. XXXIX.)

(Hips: Firm!) Knees: Bend! Stretch!

Both knees are bent simultaneously; the thighs and legs form a right-angle at the knee-joint, each knee being placed

in a line with and above the toes. The upper part of the
body is vertical and square.

(Hips: Firm!) 1. HEELS: RAISE!   ⎫ One!
               2. KNEES: BEND!   ⎪ Two!
               3. KNEES: STRETCH! ⎪ Three!
               4. HEELS: DOWN!   ⎭ Four!

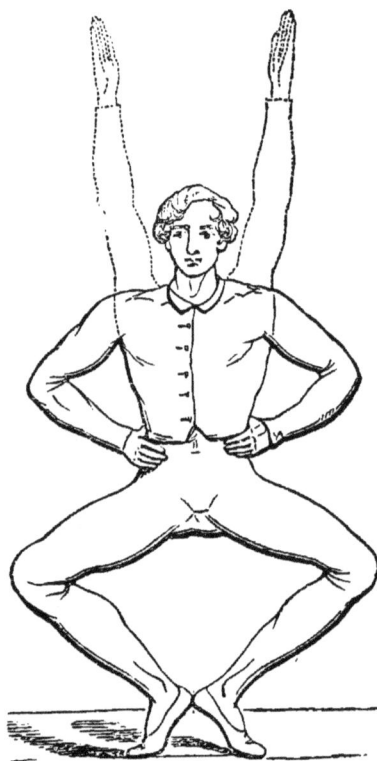

These four motions are
thus performed:—

At ONE! the heels are
raised.

At TWO! both knees are
bent, and directed outwards.

At THREE! the knees are
again stretched.

At FOUR! the heels are
placed on the floor.

This exercise is first
practised at the words of
command named before;
then, at One, Two, Three,
Four! and finally at the
words, Knees: Bend!
Stretch! which command
is given in slow time.

The exercise having been
well practised, the first
and second motions are
simultaneously done at ONE!
and at TWO! the third and

Fig. XXXIX.

fourth motions are simultaneously done; thus the knees are
bent while the heels are raised, and the knees are stretched
while the heels are placed on the floor, the stretching being
completed when the heels touch the floor.

This exercise is also useful as a balancing exercise. The
single motions must be steady, and the knees are not to be
bent beyond a right angle. If the commencing position is
FEET: OPEN! the heels touch each other during the whole
movement.

Instances of other commencing positions are—

(a) Feet sideways: Place! Knees: Bend! &c.

(b) Right (left) foot forwards (backwards): Place! Knees: Bend! &c.

(c) Right (left) foot two paces forwards: Place! Knees: Bend!

(d) Feet: Close! Knees: Bend! &c.

(e) Feet: Close! Right (left) foot forwards (backwards): Place! Knees: Bend! &c.

More advanced pupils practise the knee flexion and extension alternately, when after three, four, or five repetitions, the command HALT is given.

BENDING AND STRETCHING OF ONE KNEE IN WALK POSITION.

(See FIGS. VI. and VII.)

If the rear leg is to be bent, the words of command are—
Right (left) foot forwards: Place!

Left (right) knee: Bend! Stretch! Feet: Change! (One! Two!)

The weight of the body which is upright and square, being on the rear leg, the rear knee is bent in a right angle, while the heel is raised. The sole of the foot in front touches the floor, and the knee bends only to the extent required for placing the other knee into a right angle. After a short pause, at STRETCH! the commencing position is resumed.

At FEET: CHANGE! the right foot is drawn back, and the left placed forwards into walk position; the right knee is then bent, and stretched in the manner just described.

BENDING AND STRETCHING OF ONE KNEE IN PASS POSITION.

Right foot to the pass forwards: Place!
Front knee: Bend! Stretch!

At the first command the pass position is taken up.

At BEND! the front knee is slightly bent beyond the point of the foot, while the heel is simultaneously raised; the rear leg is well stretched, and the rear foot remains on the floor.

At STRETCH! the front foot is lowered, the heel touches the floor, the knee is in a right angle, and the body in pass position.

At FEET: CHANGE! the same movement is executed by the left knee.

ALTERNATE KNEE FLEXION IN PASS POSITION.

The right and left knees are alternately bent and stretched. The words of command are—

Right (left) foot forwards: Place!

Left knee: Bend! Stretch!

Right knee: Bend! Stretch!

These alternate movements are continued at LEFT! RIGHT! LEFT! RIGHT! till HALT is given.

At FEET: CHANGE! and ONE! both feet are placed in the commencing position; at TWO! the left (right) foot is placed in pass position; then,

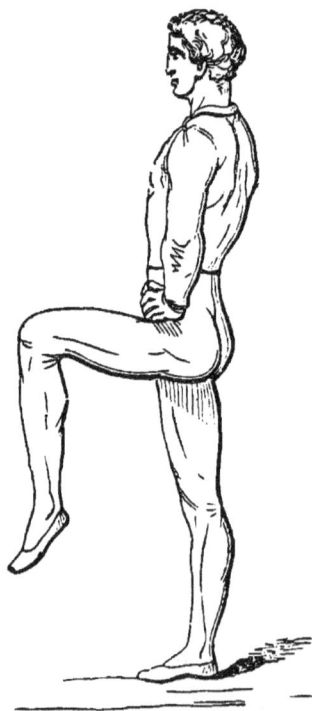

Fig. XL.

Right knee: Bend! Stretch! (One! Two! One! Two!)

Left knee: Bend! Stretch! (One! Two! One! Two!)

For those who are more advanced, the order is—

Right and left knee alternately: Bend! Stretch! Halt!

RAISING OF THE KNEE.

HIPS: FIRM! RIGHT (LEFT) KNEE: RAISE! DOWNWARDS: STRETCH!

LEFT (RIGHT) KNEE: RAISE! DOWNWARDS: STRETCH!

(Or, Feet: Change! One! Two!)

At RAISE! the right (or left) knee is quickly raised, and the foot simultaneously bent; the knee is brought into a horizontal line formed by the thigh, which is placed in the direction in which the foot is in the commencing position. The knee forms a right angle, the foot being as much as possible bent at the ankle-joint, the toes directed upwards.

At FEET: CHANGE! the change is done gently, the left (or right) knee is not raised before the right (or left) foot is firmly placed, and the right leg well stretched.

These motions are done at STRETCH! The upper part of the body remains immoveable and upright in the commencing position.

RAISING OF THE KNEE AND STRETCHING OF THE LEG.

Right (left) knee: Raise!
Right (left) knee forwards: Stretch! &c.

The knee having been raised, at STRETCH! the right (left) knee and foot are simultaneously stretched as far as possible in a horizontal line. The other leg is kept rigid, while supporting the erect trunk.

A similar exercise with the other knee is executed at FEET: CHANGE! At ONE! the fundamental position is resumed. At TWO! the left (right) leg is first raised upwards and then stretched in a similar way.

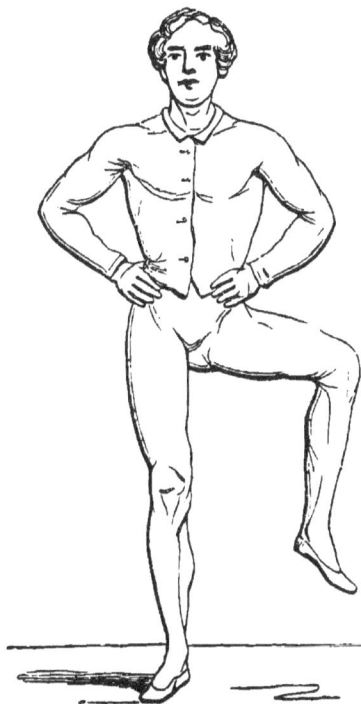

Fig. XLI.

RAISING OF THE KNEE AND MOVING IT OUTWARDS.

(FIG. XLI.)

This exercise is done at (Hips: Firm!) Knee: Raise!
KNEE OUTWARDS: MOVE!

At KNEE FORWARDS: MOVE! and FOOT: DOWN! the commencing position is resumed .

RAISING OF THE LEG.

The leg can be raised either forwards, sideways, or backwards, and the combination of these three movements forms the rotation outwards.

(Hips: Firm!) Right (left) leg forwards (sideways, backwards): Raise! Down!

At RAISE! the right (left) leg being firmly stretched, is raised forwards (sideways, or backwards.) The upper part of the body remains erect, with Hips: Firm!

At DOWN! the raised leg is slowly placed into the fundamental position.

At LEG: CHANGE! a similar exercise with the left (right) leg is done.

RAISING OF THE LEGS IN QUICK TIME, AND IN DIFFERENT DIRECTIONS,
WITH CHANGE OF LEGS.

(Hips: Firm!) Right leg forwards: Raise! Down!
Left leg sideways: Raise! Down!
Leg alternately forwards and sideways: Raise!
(One! Two!) or (Left! Right!) Down!
Leg alternately forwards and backwards: Raise!

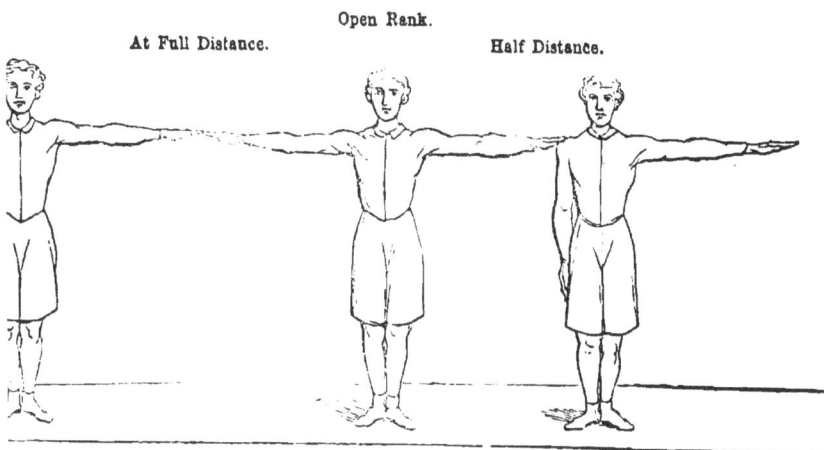

Open Rank.

At Full Distance.   Half Distance.

Fig. II.

The words of command are, *Fall in* in Rank; Half a Distance to the left (right) March! At the word March all the pupils, with the exception of the first (on the right) march in small steps to the left, sideways till the right (left) horizontally-stretched arm touches the left (right) shoulder of the neighbour on the right (left). If the order is given *Full Distance to the Left* (right) *March!* the first pupil on the right raises the left arm, all the others raise both arms, and the last raises only the right arm, while they are marching in slow paces to the left.

FORMATION IN FILE.   Fig. III.

A File Three Deep.

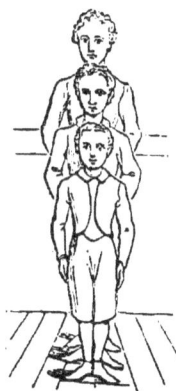

Open_File.

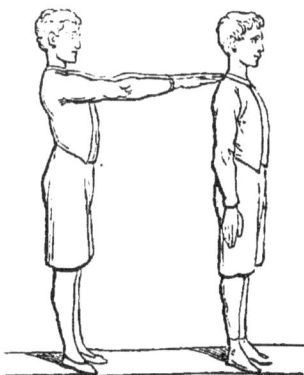

The pupils are placed one behind the other in a row, the shortest in front, and the tallest at the back. When the word Open File is given, it means that the pupils stand at half distance from each other, as seen in Fig. IV.

Fig. III.

Fig. IV.

**Three Close Ranks, or Three Files
Three Deep.**

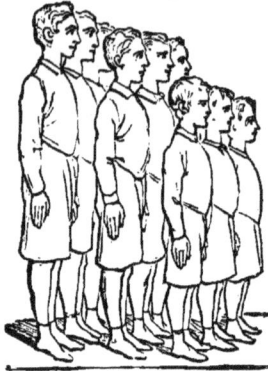

Fig. V.

Fig. V. shows the formation of nine pupils placed in *three ranks*, one behind the other, but can also represent *three files* three deep.

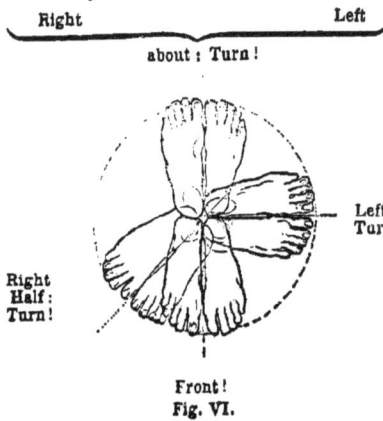

Right   Left

about : Turn!

Right
Half:
Turn!

Left:
Turn!

Front!
Fig. VI.

Fig. VI. shows how the feet are placed in *close position* in front, further in right half turn, in left turn, and in about turn. The movement of turning with the feet is done on the heels, but can also be done, as in military exercise, by placing one heel behind the other, which is done at the word *Right* (or Left), Turn! the middle of one foot is placed to the heel of the other when the word *Right* (or Left) *about* ! Turn ! is given.

Clapping of Hands.

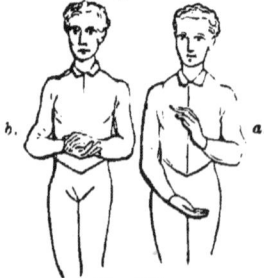

b.   a.

Fig. VII.

CLAPPING OF HANDS.

Is used for the purpose of marking time, see Fig. VII., *a*. is preparing for the clapping and *b*. is the action done at the words, Hands ! Clap !

CHANGE OF FORMATION.

If a rank formation is to be changed into file, the order is—
To the Right (or left) turn! Fig. VIII a. shows the pupils standing in close rank, and facing the teacher (the half circular line means the chest), in b. the back is turned towards the teacher, c. shows two file formations, in one, the pupils have their right and the other their left side, turned towards the teacher.

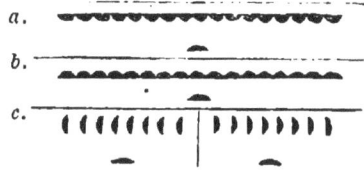

Fig. VIII.

Fig. IX a. the pupils are placed in file, form a right angle, and while marching continue forming right angles.

In b. they form an oval line.
In c. zig-zag lines.
In d. serpentine lines.

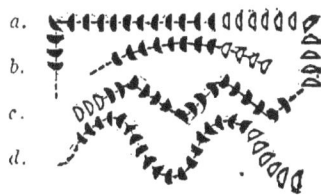

Fig. IX.

Fig. X. a. the pupils marching in single file, form a parallelogram.
b. A triangle.
c. A circle.
d. The figure 8.
e. A snail with concentric rings.

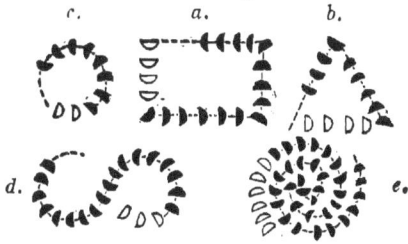

Fig. X.

Fig. XI., the pupils marching in single file are divided into two parts, each part marching first in a right angle, then form half a circle, and finally a circle.

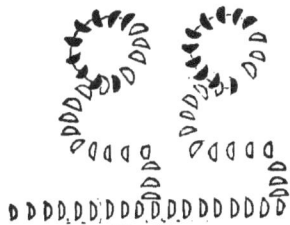

Fig. XI.

Fig. XII. Pupils being divided into two sections, march from a. and a'. in single file, one section to the right, the other to the left, forming a parallelogram till they meet at b. and b'. when they march in double file to c. and continue their counter-march, i.e., a march in which the pupils move in parallel lines. as seen in the figure.

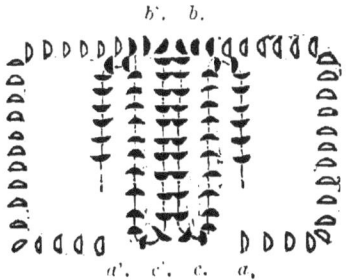

Fig. XII.

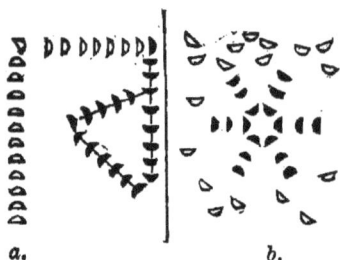

Fig. XIII. *a*. pupils marching in single file, change the rectangular figure into a triangular one. In *b*. 18 pupils are ordered to form a star with six branches each consisting of three pupils, for which purpose, the words of command would be, Fall in: in File: Tell off in Threes: Form a star!

Fig. XIII.

CHANGE OF SINGLE INTO DOUBLE FILE

Is shown in Fig. XIV. The pupils march from *a*. in single file to *b*. and turn to the right at *c*. where they again turn to the right and proceed to form the first file, while every alternate pupil continues towards *d*. where the second single file, parallel to the first, is formed.

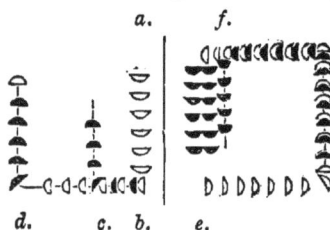

From Fig. XIV. *e*. the pupils march in single file, turn to the left, form two right angles, and turning again to the left at *f*. advance in double file.

Fig. XIV.

TELLING OFF.

When the teacher wishes to divide the pupils placed in rank or file in sections of two, three, four, or more, his word of command will be " *Tell off: in (twos), (threes), (fours),*" &c., the first pupil on the right or left of the rank, or the first or last in file calls out *one!* the second *two!* the third *three!* if they are to be divided in sections of three. The fourth calls out *one!* the fifth *two!* the sixth *three!* the seventh *one!* and so on.

In Fig. XV. *a*. the pupils being placed in rank, are ordered to tell off in sections of three; the numbers placed before each pupil are those which each has to name.

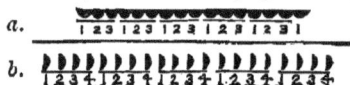

Fig. XV.

Fig. XV. *b*. the pupils placed in single file are to be divided in sections of four—when the word " *tell off: in* fours!" is given the last calls out " *one*," and the others continue to call out the numbers placed in the engraving near their *right.*

In Fig. XVI. *a*. the pupils have been told off in twos—the numbers *two* advanced two or three steps, and thus two open ranks have been formed.

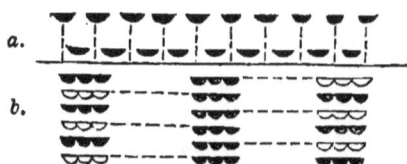

b. shows that 18 pupils divided in six sections of three—half of them placed on the right, the others on the left—

Fig. XVI.

form after marching sideways towards each other, a column of six

Fig. XVII. shows that pupils in a single file are told off in *a.* twos, *b.* and *c.* threes, *d.* and *d'.* fours, *e.* fives, and how they form (after advancing either to the left or right) a rank consisting of as many pupils as they have been told off.

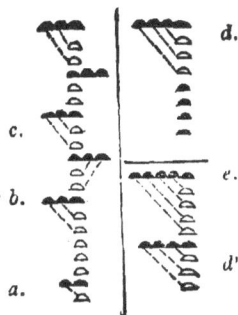

Fig. XVII.

CHANGE OF SINGLE INTO DOUBLE AND TRIPLE FILE

Is seen in Fig. XVIII. The pupils march from *a.* in single file, turn at *b.* to the left, form, after turning to the left at *c.* a double file, advance to *d.* turn to the right and continue in single file till *e.* where they turn to the right, advance in triple file, turn at *f.* to the left, advance towards *g.* where they change, after having turned to the left into a double file, continue to march forward, turn at *h.* and after another turn to the right, they continue in single file.

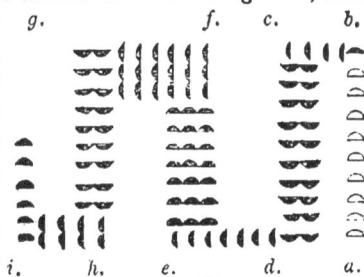

Fig. XVIII.

"Break : rank !" or "Break : file !" is the order given when the pupils placed in rank or file are to leave off this formation. Fig. XIX. *a.* shows the breaking of double close rank, *b.* of double file, *c.* of *three ranks*, each consisting of a section of five pupils, *d.* of a triple file.

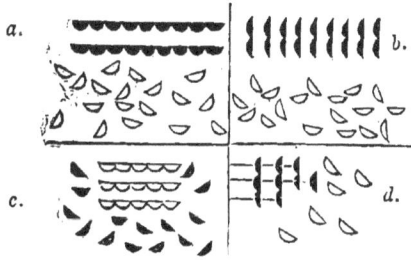

Fig. XIX.

Fig. XX. shows the breaking of rank and file, as well as the formation of 16 pupils divided in sections of four, each of the sections having another formation, the teacher represented by the arger black half-circle, facing the pupils.

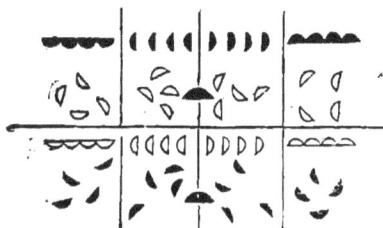

Fig. XX.

WHEELING

Is a movement of a section round a fixed point, thus a section of three pupils standing in close rank can wheel round each of the three.

Fig. XXI. *a*. represents the wheeling *to the left* of three pupils, the first on the left of the rank turns to the left on the spot on which he stands, while the second and third march till they are in the same line as the first; at the word " *to the right wheel :* march!" the pupil who is the first on the right of the rank turns on the spot to the right, at *a'*. while the second and third remaining in close rank march till they are in a line with the first, as seen in the rank formed *b*. by the three dark spots. Fig. XXI. *b*. represents seven pupils standing in close rank, they are ordered to "wheel on the centre to the right: march!" the fourth pupil forming the centre turns to *the right* on the spot where he stands, the three pupils on the left of the centre march forwards, the three others march backwards till they are in the line *c*, which is perpendicular to the previous *b*. If the order " *To the right: wheel!*" is given three times more, the pupils return into their original positions, and a whole wheel has been formed.

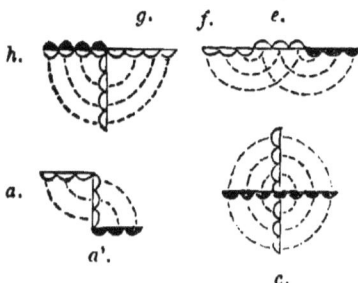

Fig. XXI.

d. Fig. XXI. shows a rank of three pupils wheeling to the *right* about till they are in *e*., or the rank of *f*. is wheeling to the *left about* and arrive also at *e*., thus in "*wheel: about!*" half a circle is formed.

A section of four is wheeling *to the right and right about* from *g*. to *h*., Fig. XXI.

Fig. XXII. represents the formation of a square by 16 pupils who are first divided in two sections of eight, later in four sections of four, and at the order of wheeling form the square.

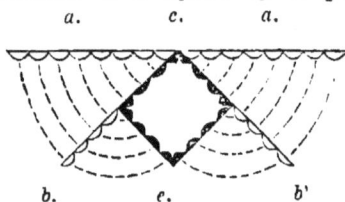

The words of command are :
" Fall in : close rank!"
" Tell off in eights!"
Section on the right to the left ⎱ *wheel.*
    ,,   ,,   left   ,,   right ⎰

Fig. XXII.

March! at this word the sections march till they arrive in *b. b'.* where a right angle is formed in *c*, at the word *halt!*

Tell off in fours.

Sections forming right angle stop, the other two sections wheel one to the left the other to the right at the word *march!* and stop when the angle *e*. is formed at the word *halt!*

Free Exercises with Assistance or Resistance.

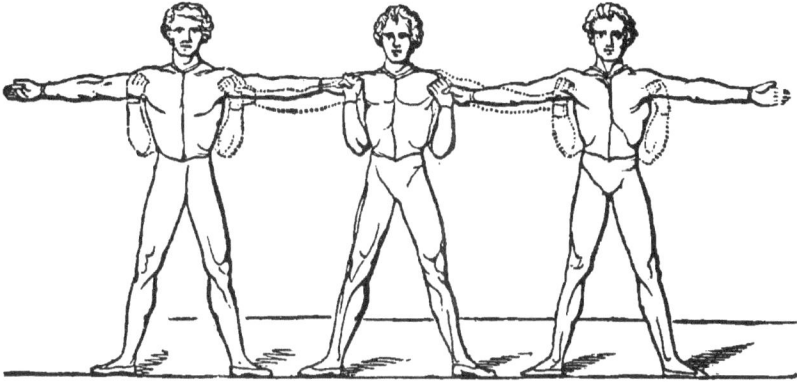

Fig. XXIII.

These exercises are more difficult, and the pupils must be well trained in the previous exercises before assistance is given or resistance can be used. Fig. XXIII. is only to serve as an instance of the manner this is done.

Three pupils are standing in stride position, the second has the forearms in *upwards: bend!* position, while the first and third are taking hold of his hands. They may offer him some resistance, while he is to stretch the arms sideways, or they may assist him in doing the desired movement which is shown by the dotted lines *

Combination of Marching and Running.

The following is an example of one section marching in line, while the other section is running.

The Weaver's Run.—Fig. XXIV. This exercise is done by two sections, the *ones* (a. b. c. d.) stand in a chain; that is, they take hold of each other's hands, with distance in front; the *twos* (a. b. c.) stand in a row one after the other, sideways with regard to the *ones*, and a few paces in advance. At the word "Weaver's run: march!" the *ones* walk abreast in chain walk straight forwards at quick step; the *twos* at the same moment begin the short run in a transversal direction, passing the front of the *ones*, when the last *two* (that is c.) comes in front of the interval between a. and b., and the other *twos* in front of the other intervals, they turn sharply and

---

* NOTE.—Fig. XXIII and Fig. XXIV are taken from the 2nd edition of Dr. Roths' translation of Rothsteins' Gymnastic Free Exercises of Ling, a little book specially recommended to teachers who wish to know more on this subject.

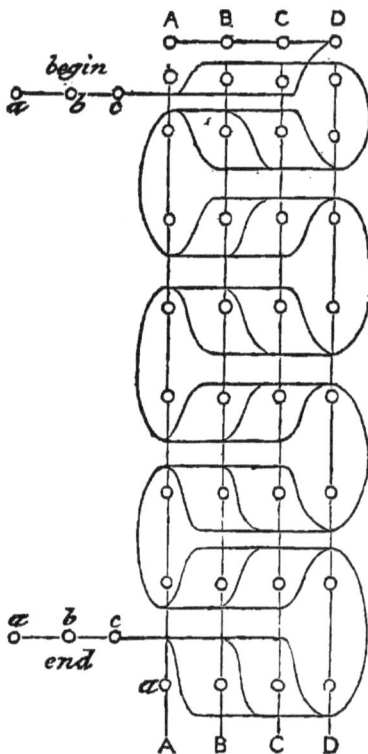

Fig. XXIV.

run round and come in front.

pass between A. B. C. D. the *ones* breaking the chain for a moment; as soon as they have passed the intervals, they turn behind A. B. C. D., and run round D, so as to come once more in front of A. B. C. D.; they then pass through the same intervals, and then, turning sharply, pass round A. and come once more in front. When this has been done five to ten times (according to the space at disposal), the sections change in the movements. To do this exercise with one section, there must not be less than seven persons, and not more than from 20 to 24; and they must be divided in such a way that those who advance straight on, should consist of one more than the others, that there may be an interval for each *two*. That the interval passage may be done uniformly, the *ones* must for several seconds *mark time** with the feet, while the others

---

* This signifies that the feet are lifted in time, without moving from the spot.

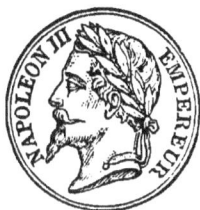

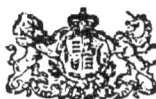

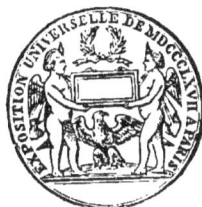

EDUCATIONAL PUBLICATIONS

OF

A. N. MYERS & CO.,

15, BERNERS STREET, OXFORD STREET, LONDON, W.

	£	s.	d.
EMBOSSED ATLAS, accurately executed in Relief and Colours, illustrating clearly the Physical features of the Earth. Seven Maps—The World, Europe, Asia, Africa, South America, North America, Australia and Polynesia; neatly mounted and varnished; in frames 11 by 9 inches; accompanied by a corresponding series of Maps printed in colours in accordance with the Political divisions. The whole enclosed in a neat box	0	15	0
'HE MANUFACTURE OF A NEEDLE. An interesting account of its History and Manufacture, from the earliest ages to the present time, by Charles Tomlinson; accompanied by a card of Specimens illustrating the various Stages of Progress, from the Rough Metal to the Finished Article . . . . In cloth case	0	1	6
THE MANUFACTURE OF A STEEL PEN, by Charles Tomlinson. Uniform with the above	0	1	6
THE MANUFACTURE OF A PIN, by Charles Tomlinson, ditto . .	0	1	6
THE MANUFACTURE OF PAPER, by Charles Tomlinson; accompanied by a book of Specimens of the Principal Kinds of Paper. In cloth case .	0	1	6
DOLLY'S DRESSMAKER; a Gift for Young Ladies. Comprising Coloured Patterns, and 12 Lithographed Sheets of Pattern Outlines for DOLLS' DRESSES of all kinds, with descriptive letter-press, translated from the German of Frederika Lesser, by Madame de Chatelain; in a portfolio. Series I., II., and III. Each Series complete in itself	0	2	0

DOLLS to suit the above in size, of various kinds and prices.

	£	s.	d.
EXERCISES IN COLOURING WITH RHYMES. No. 1, PRETTY PICTURES; No. 2, THE FAIR. Each Book contains 8 Coloured Pictures with English Rhymes underneath, and side by side the uncoloured counterparts with a German Version of the Rhymes	0	0	6
EXERCISES IN COLOURING—GEOMETRICAL TERMS ILLUSTRATED BY COMMON OBJECTS. Two Parts, each containing 16 quarter-page Coloured Illustrations, with uncoloured counterparts side by side. Per Part	0	0	6

A large variety of other Subjects of EXERCISES IN COLOURING, *may be had uniform with the above.*

	£	s.	d.
HERMES' DRAWING SCHOOL, in 500 Parts, comprising First Lessons, Landscapes, Flowers and Fruits, Arabesques, Studies from Still Life, Animals, the Human Form, Geometrical and Architectural Drawing. Each Part, Demy 8vo., with 6 Plates	0	0	8